BALANCE EXERCISE

FOR SENIORS

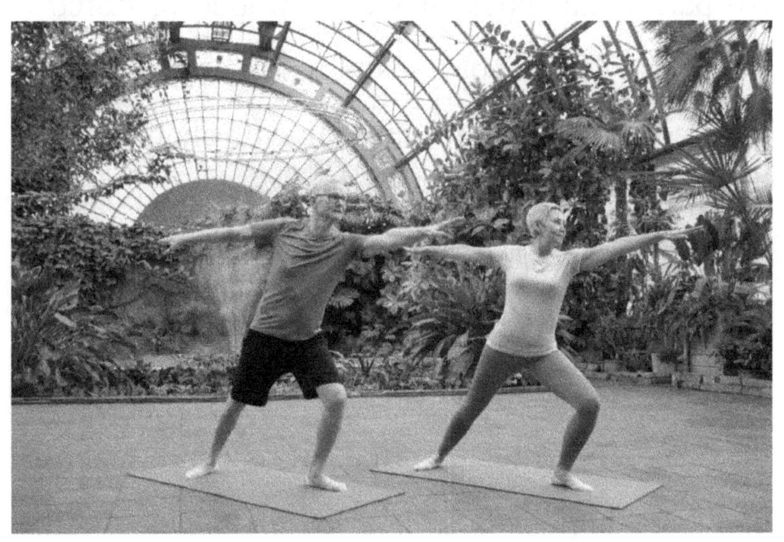

ACHIEVING OPTIMAL BALANCE AND STABILITY WITH AGE APPROPRIATE EXERCISES

KAREN WALDROP

Table of Content

CHAPTER 6: STRENGTH TRAINING FOR SENIORS

CHAPTER 12: STAYING MOTIVATED

CONCLUSION

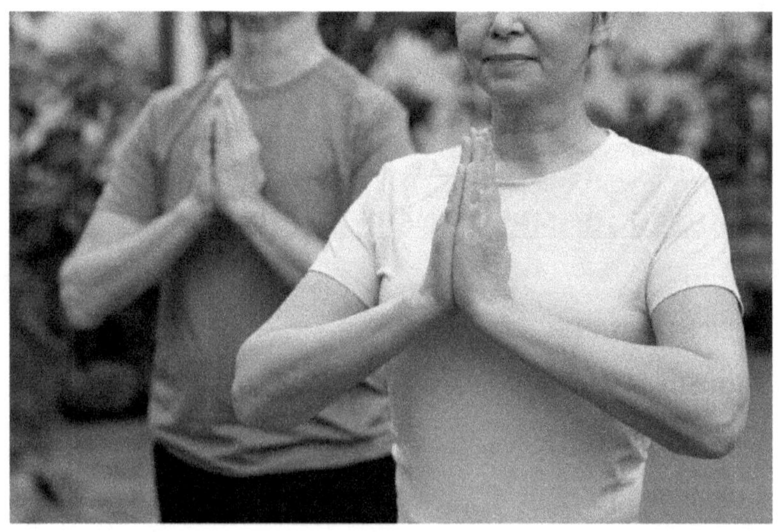

Introduction

David, a sixty-year-old man, has struggled with health issues for a while. Although he had always been active, his joints had recently become stiff, making it difficult for him to move.

On one occasion, while on a stroll, he saw his neighbor—a physical therapist and a writer—in her nursery. He approached her, and they started joking about it. When she asked about his financial situation, he revealed his troubles with adaptability.

Before telling him about her book, Balance Exercise for seniors, she made a kind gesture to him. She said that by doing the activities in the book, David and other individuals like him may enhance their general wellness.

David was fascinated and inquired about buying the book. She handed him a copy and immediately agreed.

Over the following weeks, David completed the exercises in the book and was astounded by the results. His joints were much more adaptive, he had more energy, and he could walk without pain.

He was receptive to the advice and book recommendations from his neighbor. He thanked her enthusiastically and pledged to keep in contact.

David could continue his complete workout regimen since his health had substantially advanced. He could now spend more time with his friends and family and walk in the leisure area.

He was incredibly grateful for his neighbor's assistance and the book she had written, which radically altered his life. He could now enjoy life and continue to be active for the vast majority of his remaining years.

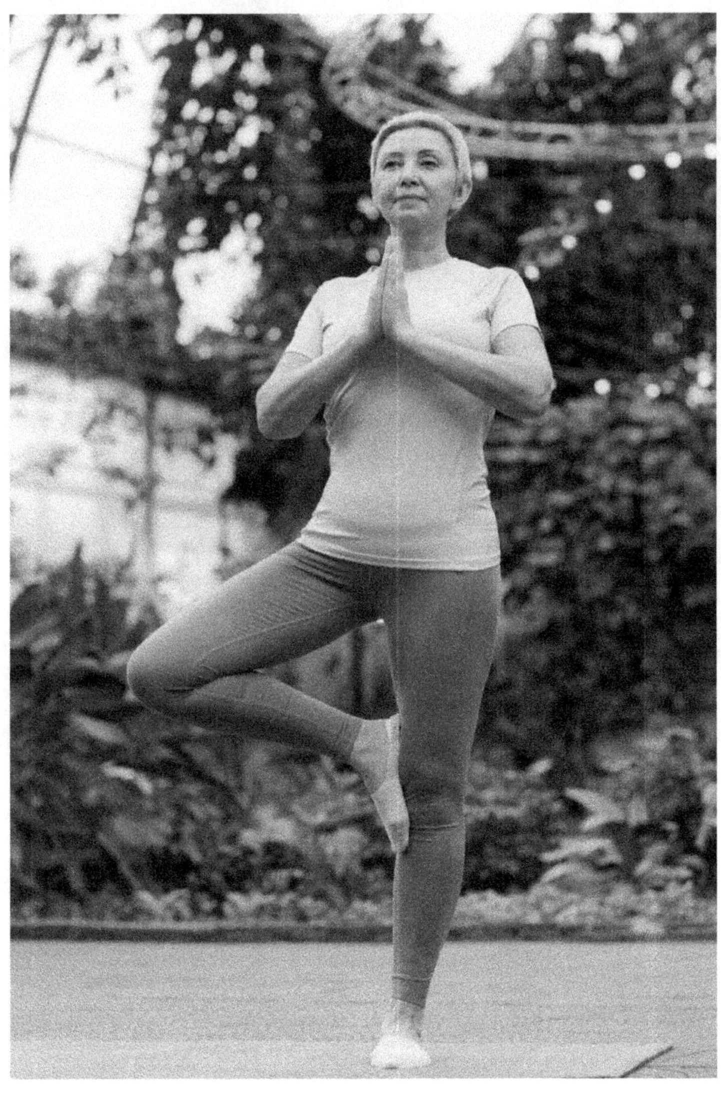

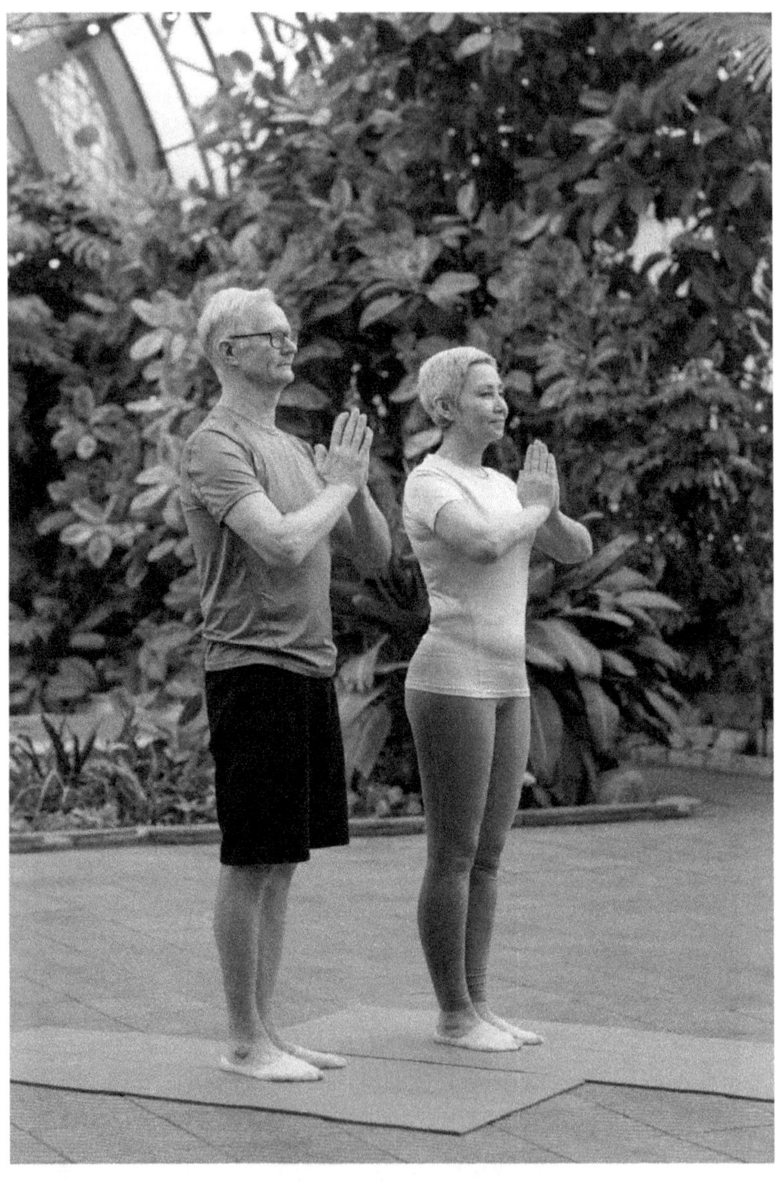

Chapter 1: Aging and Exercise

It's a common perception that aging and exercise are related issues. Our bodies naturally weaken and become more prone to disease and injury as we age, so it's essential to maintain a healthy lifestyle that includes regular exercise. Regardless of age, practice may support maintaining and enhancing one's physical and mental health.

For healthy aging, exercise offers several advantages. Additionally, it may lower the chance of contracting conditions like osteoporosis, heart disease, and diabetes by maintaining the strength and flexibility of the body's muscles, bones, and joints. Along with lowering stress levels, boosting mood, and boosting energy, exercise may also aid in preserving cognitive function.

Adapting exercise to a person's requirements is possible. Starting gently and gradually increasing the intensity and length of activity over time is crucial for people just starting an exercise regimen.

Seniors should focus on strength training to preserve muscle mass and reduce the risk of falling. Free weights, weight machines, and resistance bands should be used for strength training. Walking, jogging, or swimming are all examples of aerobic activities beneficial for cardiovascular health.

For seniors, balance exercises are extremely crucial since they may lower the chance of falling. Yoga, tai chi, and balancing boards are just a few workouts that improve balance. A fitness program should include stretching, weight training, aerobics, and balancing exercises as just a few examples.

To assist the body in recovering from exercise, it is crucial to include rest days in an exercise regimen. For the body to perform at its best, consuming a balanced diet and keeping hydrated is also critical. For good aging, exercise is crucial. As well as lowering the chance of contracting certain illnesses, it may assist in maintaining and even enhancing physical and mental well-being.

Stretching, weight training, aerobics, and balancing exercises are just a few of the activities that should be included in an exercise program specifically designed to meet the requirements of each person. Incorporating rest days, staying hydrated, and eating a balanced diet are also crucial. Regardless of age, seniors may maintain physical and mental fitness with the correct exercise regimen.

Assessing Your Current Balance as a senior

Evaluating your existing balance as a senior is an essential first step to fully comprehending your physical capabilities and pinpointing any areas needing development. Strength, coordination, flexibility, and sensory perception work together to create balance a complicated process that may alter as you age.

Start by watching your daily activities to determine your current balance. Keep track of any problems you have walking, getting out of a chair, or staying stable on uneven ground. These observations may provide insightful information about possible balance problems.

Next, test your stability with a few easy balancing exercises. The "single-leg stand," which involves standing on one leg and timing how long you can keep your balance, is a typical test. The "tandem stand," which requires standing heel to toe with one foot in front of the other, is an additional test. It would help if you watched for any swaying, loss of balance, or difficulty maintaining the postures.

Try timing how long it takes to get up from a chair, walk a short distance, turn around, and get back down. It is known as the "get up and go" test. Your general mobility, transitional balance, and coordination are all evaluated by this exam.

Speak with a senior care expert in the medical field, such as a physical therapist. They can conduct more thorough evaluations, including the Timed Up and Go exam or the Berg Balance Scale. These evaluations provide precise measures and support identifying specific areas that need improvement.

By evaluating your current balance, you may learn a lot about your physical capabilities and any prospective problem areas. You may use it to measure your progress and customize your balancing training program to target certain deficiencies or restrictions. Remember that particular exercises and practice may help you improve your balance, and frequent evaluations can help you track your development and maintain your stability as you age.

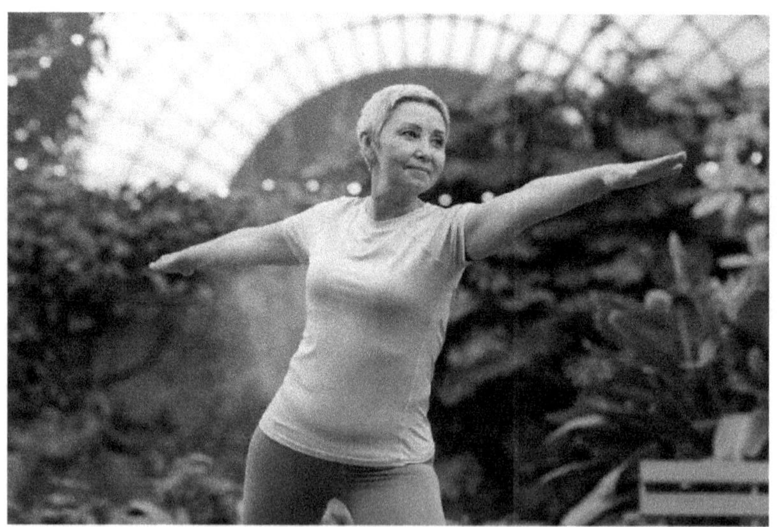

Chapter 2: Benefits of Exercise for seniors

Exercise has several advantages for seniors that increase general health, happiness, and lifespan. The following are some significant advantages of training, especially for seniors:

Improved Physical Health: Regular exercise benefits seniors' physical health in several ways. It may improve flexibility, balance, muscular strength, cardiovascular fitness, and general mobility. These advantages help lower the risk of fractures, falls, and chronic illnesses, including diabetes, heart disease, and osteoporosis.

Increased Independence: Exercise helps seniors keep their independence and efficiently carry out everyday tasks by enhancing strength, endurance, and flexibility. It involves walking, stair climbing, carrying groceries, and keeping one's self-clean.

Maintaining independence improves life satisfaction and promotes independence.

Improved Cognitive Performance: Exercise enhances the brain's health and cognitive performance. Seniors' memory, focus, and executive abilities may be improved. Regular exercise triggers the production of neurotrophic substances like brain-derived neurotrophic factor (BDNF), which support the growth and development of neurons and improve cognitive function.

The benefits of exercise for mental health are substantial.

Endorphins, or "feel-good" hormones, are released due to movement. These chemicals have antidepressant and anti anxiety effects as well as mood-improving and general mental health benefits. Seniors may naturally and quickly control and lower their risk of mental health disorders by exercising regularly.

Social Engagement: Seniors who participate in exercise activities like walking clubs or group fitness programs have possibilities for social engagement. It encourages connections and emotional support while fostering community and preventing social isolation. Exercise's social component has a favorable effect on both mental health and general well-being.

Regular exercise is essential for avoiding and controlling several chronic illnesses often brought on by aging. It helps manage blood pressure, lowers the risk of heart disease and stroke, enhances insulin sensitivity, and improves blood sugar control. In addition, exercise may aid in managing respiratory infections, chronic discomfort, and rheumatoid arthritis.

 Insomnia and interrupted sleep are common sleep disorders among seniors. Regular exercise may lengthen and increase the quality of sleep. Physical activity encourages the release of brain chemicals like serotonin, which control sleep cycles and help seniors have more peaceful and restorative sleep.

Exercise has a natural calming impact that helps elderly cope with stress's physical and mental repercussions. Exercise increases endorphin synthesis, which lowers cortisol levels and other stress chemicals. Exercises regimens give seniors time to think about themselves, let off steam, and enhance stress management.

Increased lifespan and a decreased risk of early death in seniors have been related to regular exercise. Exercise may significantly contribute to a longer and better life by enhancing general health, avoiding chronic illnesses, and enhancing functional capacities.

Seniors who exercise will ultimately live longer and with a more excellent quality of life. They can keep their freedom, participate in their hobbies, encounter fewer health restrictions, and have higher physical and emotional well-being. Long into one's senior years, regular exercise encourages an active and meaningful existence.

Exercise helps elders in various ways, including promoting physical health, emotional health, cognitive function, and overall quality of life. Seniors may improve their health and benefit from an active lifestyle by including regular exercise in their daily activities.

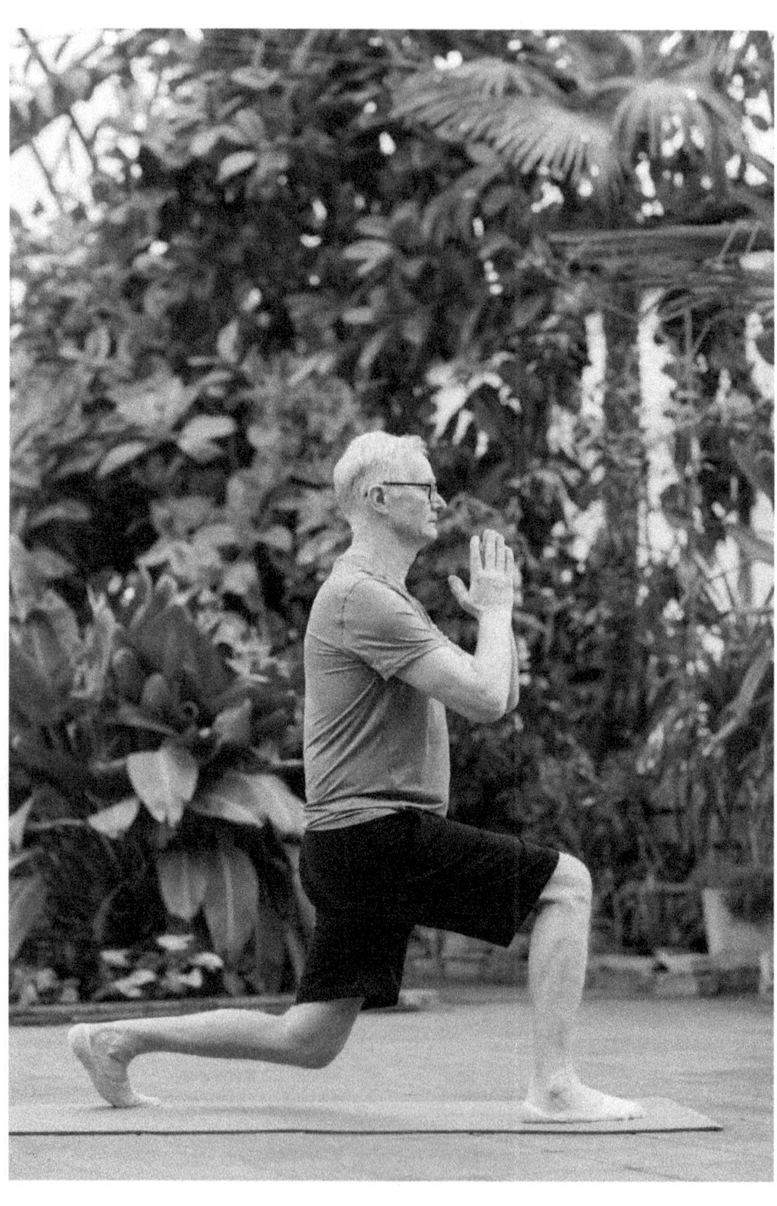

Chapter 3: Types of Exercise for seniors

Seniors may participate in various activities to enhance their general health, flexibility, and balance. Here are a few exercises that are very good for seniors:

Aerobic Exercise

Brisk Walking: is a low-impact activity that is simple to include in regular schedules. The practice strengthens both the cardiovascular system and the leg muscles.

Swimming: Water activities are easy on the joints and provide the whole body with a workout, boosting muscular strength and cardiovascular fitness.

Cycling:

- Cycling on a stationary cycle or outside may enhance joint mobility, leg strength, and cardiovascular health.

Strength training

- Resistance bands may increase strength without placing undue strain on the joints. It can be used for various workouts that target specific muscle areas.

- Weight machines are a safe way for seniors to increase their strength and muscular tone at gyms and fitness facilities.

- Exercises that utilize your body weight as resistance, such as squats, lunges, push-ups, and planks, help you gain strength and stability.

Flexibility and Balance Exercises

Yoga: Yoga includes gentle movements, stretches, and breathing techniques to improve flexibility, balance, and relaxation.

Tai Chi: This traditional Chinese exercise involves gentle, fluid motions that increase balance, coordination, and strength while encouraging relaxation and serenity.

Pilates: Pilates emphasizes regulated movements to build core strength, flexibility, and balance, which improve posture and stability in general.

Low-impact workouts

Exercises in a chair, such as leg lifts, arm curls, and seated marching, are an option for seniors with restricted mobility.

Low-Impact Aerobics: Senior-friendly low-impact aerobic programs and exercise DVDs promote cardiovascular health without putting undue strain on the joints.

As was already said, Tai Chi is a moderate workout that may benefit seniors of all fitness levels.

Exercises for Stability and Balance

Standing Leg Lifts: Raising the other leg behind or to the side while standing on one leg may strengthen your legs and enhance your balance.

Walking with one heel in front of the other's toes is known as a heel-to-toe walk, which may aid balance and coordination.

Stability balls or balancing boards: These exercises may test your stability and balance while strengthening your core and improving your coordination.

Before beginning any new exercise program, seniors must speak with their healthcare doctors or fitness expert. They may provide individualized advice while considering each person's degree of fitness, medical issues, and limits. Additionally, it's crucial to begin carefully, pay attention to your body, and gradually increase the length and intensity of your workouts over time.

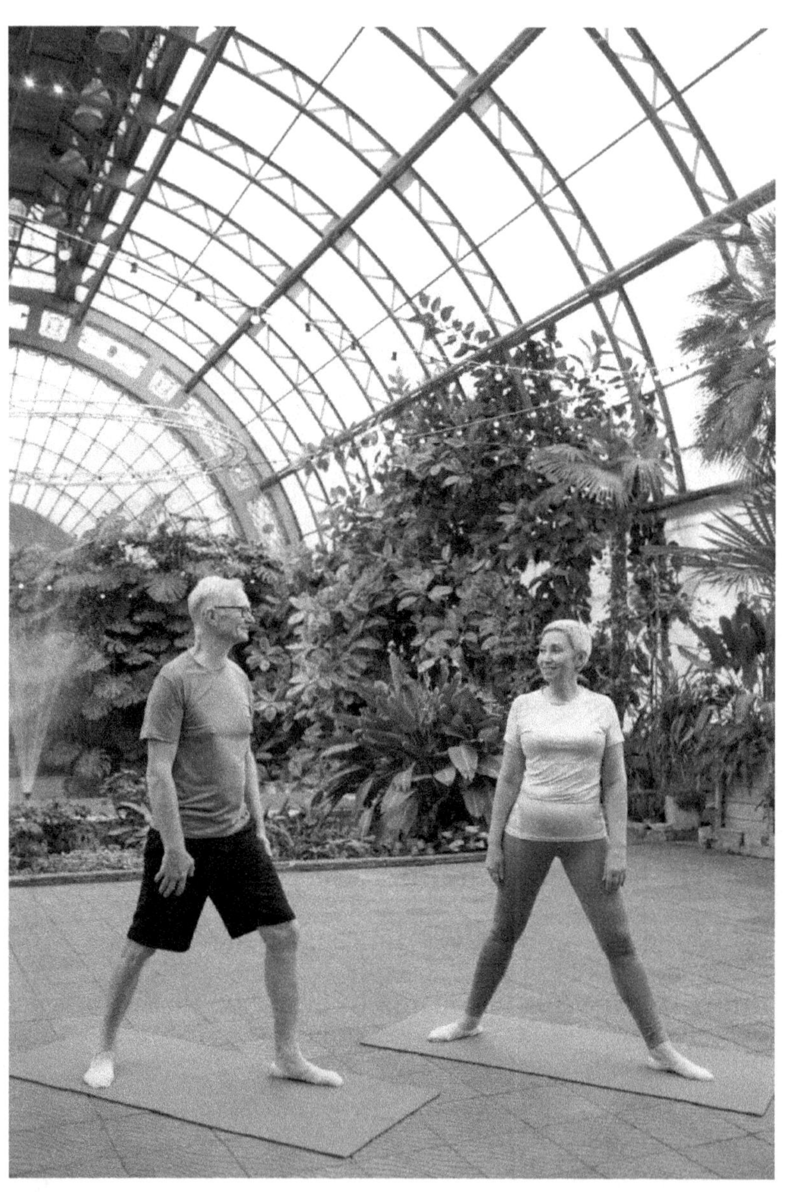

Chapter 4: Getting Started with Exercise

Seniors may improve their general health, preserve their independence, and improve their quality of life by starting an exercise regimen. To get created safely and successfully, follow these steps:

Consult Your Healthcare Provider: It's essential to speak with your healthcare provider before starting any new fitness regimen, particularly if you have any current medical issues or worries. They may provide insightful advice and guarantee that exercising is secure and appropriate for your requirements.

Determine what you want to accomplish with your fitness program and set realistic goals. Setting realistic and attainable objectives can keep you motivated and focused, whether you aim to manage a particular health condition, increase strength, increase flexibility, or improve cardiovascular fitness.

Start Slowly and Advance progressively: As your level of fitness increases, progressively increase the intensity, length, and complexity of your workouts. This strategy aids injury prevention and enables your body to adjust to exercise demands.

Pick Interests You Enjoy:

Choose workouts that you like and are compatible with your interests and skills. Your exercises will become more pleasurable and durable as a result. Finding things you like doing can help you remain motivated, whether walking, swimming, dancing, or doing yoga.

Warm-Up and Cool-Down: Before beginning each workout session, gently warm up your muscles by stretching or walking in place. It lowers the possibility of damage while helping your body prepare for activity. Similarly, end each session with a stretch and cooling time to drop your heart rate gradually.

Include a Variety of Exercises: Mix exercises for balance, flexibility, strength, and aerobics into your regimen. It guarantees that you will benefit from a comprehensive fitness regimen. Aim for two or more days a week of strength training exercises that target the main muscle groups, coupled with at least 150 minutes of moderate-intensity aerobic activity. To prevent damage, you should pay attention to your body and alter or change your actions as necessary. Consult your healthcare practitioner if you have any unexpected symptoms or chronic discomfort.

Drink plenty of water before, during, and after exercise to keep you hydrated and nourished. Maintain a well-balanced diet with sufficient nutrients, such as protein, to aid muscle repair and general health.

Find a Supportive Environment: Consider signing up for senior-specific fitness programs or organizations. It creates a friendly and encouraging atmosphere where you meet others with similar objectives and difficulties. You may maintain your motivation and commitment to your workout regimen with the support and encouragement of others.

Be Consistent: To profit from exercise, you must be consistent. As your fitness level increases, the frequency and length of your workouts progressively increase. Even if you may only start with brief sessions, being consistent will eventually lead to fruitful outcomes.

Remember that you may always start exercising and enjoy the advantages of an active lifestyle. You may benefit from the physical, mental, and emotional benefits of regular exercise as a senior with the right coaching and a tailored strategy.

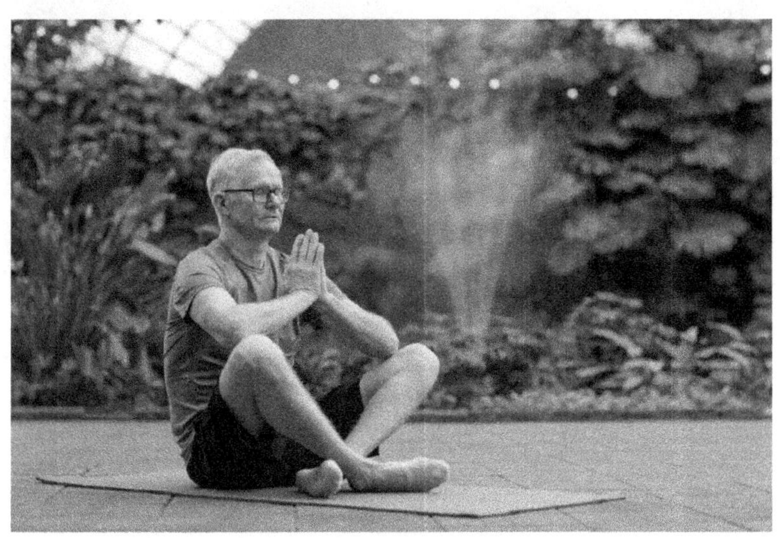

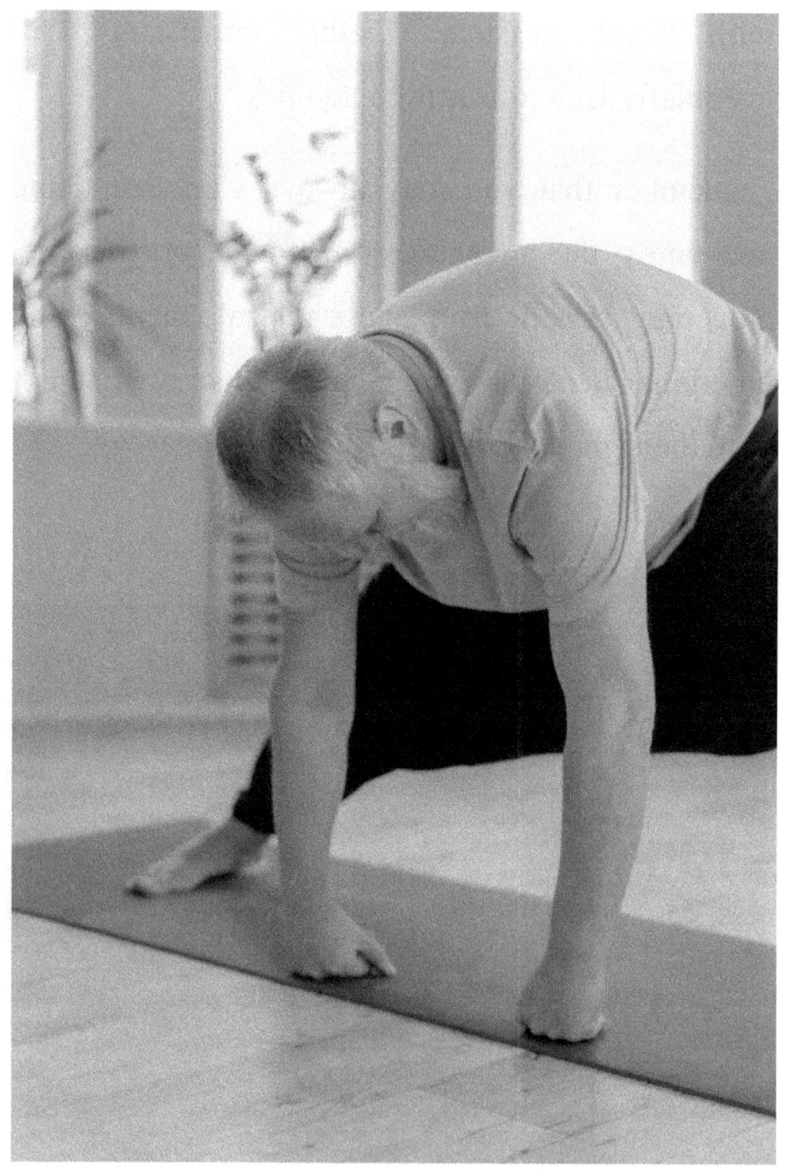

Chapter 5: Stretching Exercises for seniors

A senior's well-rounded fitness program must include stretching activities. They aid in increasing the range of motion, maintaining muscle balance, and lowering injury risk. Stretching helps improve posture, reduce muscular tension, and encourage relaxation. Here is a thorough list of stretching activities for seniors:

Neck Stretches

- Whether standing or sitting up straight, gradually bend your head to the side so your ear is closer to your shoulder.

- For 15 to 30 seconds on each side, hold the stretch.

Neck Side Stretch

- Slowly move your neck to one side while seeing over your shoulder.
- After holding for 15 to 30 seconds, switch to the other side.

Shoulder Stretches

Shoulder Rolls:

- Do ten to fifteen shoulder rolls, rolling your shoulders backward and forth in a circular manner.

Shoulder Cross Stretch:

- Stretch your shoulders by extending one arm across your chest and slowly bringing the other closer.

- Hold each position for 15–30 seconds.

Chest Stretches

Chest Opener:

- Stand close to a doorway, rest your forearms on each side of the door frame, and step forward until your chest muscles extend.

- For 15 to 30 seconds, hold.

Wall Push-Up Stretch:

- Stand facing a wall, put your hands on the wall at shoulder height, and gently lean forward until you feel your chest extend.

- For 15 to 30 seconds, hold.

Back Stretches

Spinal twist:

- While seated in a chair and putting your feet level on the floor, gradually rotate your upper body to the other side while resting your opposite palm on the outside of your thigh.

- Hold each position for 15–30 seconds.

Cat- Camel Stretch:

- Begin on your hands and knees.

- Circle your back toward the ceiling like a cat.

- Arch your back down, elevating your chest and buttocks toward the top.

- This stretch is known as the cat-camel stretch. Repeat ten to fifteen times.

Hip stretches

Hip Flexor Stretch:

- Stretch your hip flexors by lunging forward while maintaining your back knee on the floor.

- Feel the front of your hip being stretched as you slowly transfer your weight forward.

- Hold each position for 15–30 seconds.

Seated Hip Stretch:

- Hip stretches, when established, including sitting on the edge of a chair, crossing one ankle over the other knee, and gently pressing down on the lifted knee until you feel a stretch in your hip.

- Hold each position for 15–30 seconds.

Leg Stretches

Standing Calf Stretch:

- Stand close to a wall while holding onto anything solid and step back with your heel still on the ground.

- Feeling your leg muscle stretch, lean forward.

- Hold each position for 15–30 seconds.

Seated hamstring stretch:

- Lean forward.

- Reach for your toes.

- Sit on the edge of a chair while extending one leg straight in front of you.

- You should feel a stretch at the back of your leg.

- Hold each position for 15–30 seconds.

Balance and Flexibility Exercises:

Tree Pose:

- In this position, you should stand tall, transfer your weight to one foot, put the sole of your other foot on the inner thigh of the leg you are standing on, and establish your balance. Before switching sides, hold for 15 to 30 seconds.

- Stretch your quadriceps by bending one knee, standing close to a wall, or holding onto a solid surface. Then, draw your foot toward your buttocks by grabbing your ankle.

- Take a 15- to 30-second hold on each side.

Full-Body Stretches

Standing Side Bend:

- Stand tall with your feet hip-width apart to do this exercise.

- Raise one arm above, and then gently bend your upper body to the side until you feel a stretch along the side of your body.

- Hold each side for 15–30 seconds, then switch sides.

- **Full-Body Stretch:**

- Stand tall with your feet hip-width apart, raise your arms aloft, entwine your fingers, and stretch upward.

- Feel a stretch across your whole body as you lengthen your spine and reach toward the ceiling.

- Pause for 15–30 seconds.

-

Tips for Safe Stretching

Breathe:

- Throughout each stretch, take slow, deep breaths. Deeply inhale through your nose, and then gradually exhale through your mouth.

Gradual Progression:

- Begin with easy stretches and build up to more strenuous ones over time.

- Hurt might result from bouncing or jerky motions, so avoid these.

Take Note of Your Body:

- Pay attention to the cues from your body. Stretch is just enough to feel a little pull or strain but insufficient to cause discomfort.

- While discomfort is joint, acute or intense pain is uncommon.

Personalize Your Stretches:

- Concentrate on where you feel tight or constrained. Because everyone's range of motion varies, modify the stretches to meet your body's requirements.

Warm up:

- Stretching should be preceded by a short aerobic warm-up that includes brisk walking or marching in place.

- By doing so, you improve blood flow and get your muscles ready for stretching.

Stretch Both Sides:

- Always extend both sides to keep your body balanced and symmetrical.

Consistency:

- Aim to stretch at least twice or thrice weekly.

- The secret to preserving and enhancing flexibility is consistency.

Although stretching is advantageous, the extension should differ from other elements of a well-rounded fitness program, like strength training and aerobic activity. Combining these factors, you may obtain your best level of physical fitness and general well-being as a senior.

Always check with your doctor before beginning any new fitness regimen, including stretches, particularly if you have any current medical issues or worries. Depending on your particular requirements, they may provide individualized advice and direction.

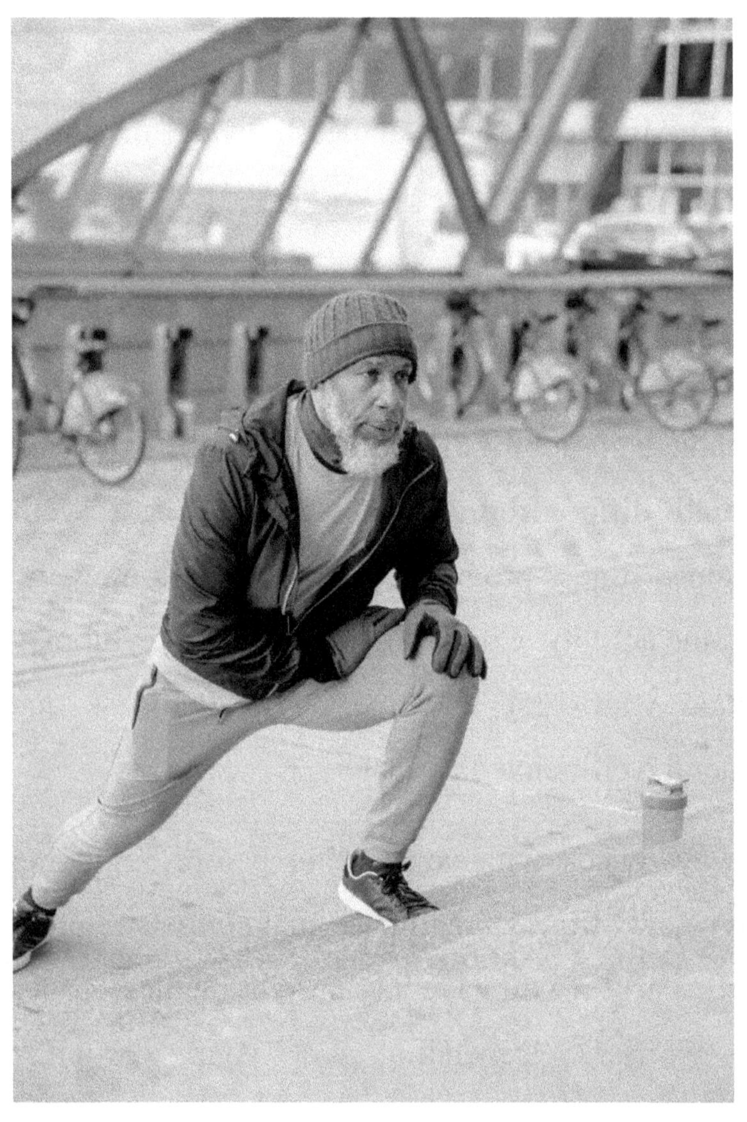

Chapter 6: Strength Training for Seniors

Weightlifting, usually called strength training, is a healthy exercise for seniors. It supports total functional independence by enhancing balance, stability, bone density, and muscular strength. Frequent strength training can facilitate a healthier, more active lifestyle. Here, you will find a comprehensive manual on strength training for seniors.

Benefits of Strength Training for seniors

- Strength exercise helps maintain and develop muscular mass, essential for preserving strength and functional skills as we age.

- Resistance training encourages bone development, which lowers the risk of osteoporosis and fractures and improves bone health.

- Enhanced Metabolism: Strength training may aid in boosting metabolism, supporting a healthy weight control approach.

- Seniors may enhance their balance and stability by strengthening their muscles, especially those in their lower bodies and core, lowering their chance of falling.

- Enhanced Joint Function: Muscles surrounding the joints are supported and protected when stronger, which helps with arthritis-related pain and stiffness.

- Strength exercise generates endorphins, which boosts mood and, lowers the risk of sadness and anxiety—improves Mental Well-Being.

Seniors' Recommended Exercises

Squats

- Stand with your feet hip-width apart, bend your knees and hips to lower your body, and then push yourself back up to the starting position.

- Squats bolster the lower body's strength, particularly the thighs, hips, and buttocks.

Lunges

- Step forward on one leg and make a lunge by bending both knees until they are at a 90-degree angle.

- Reposition yourself so that you are where you were when you started.

- Rushes exercise the quadriceps, hamstrings, and glutes.

Chest press

- Holding weights or resistance bands at chest level do a chest press while seated or lying on a bench, stability ball, or flat surface.

- The chest, shoulders, and triceps are strengthened through chest pushes.

Seated Row

- While sitting on a bench, stability ball, or flat surface, pull weights or resistance bands toward your body while pushing your shoulder blades together.

- Rowing, while seated, works the biceps and upper back.

Leg press

- Lie on a leg press machine with your feet on the footplate.

- Push the footplate away by spreading your legs.

- Return to the beginning position.

- The quadriceps, hamstrings, and glutes are all worked out with leg presses.

Shoulder Press

- Stand or sit while holding weights or resistance bands at shoulder level, then push them above until you fully stretch your arms.

- Shoulder presses bolster the upper arms and shoulders.

Triceps dips

- Bend your elbows to bring your body down, and then raise it until your arms are straight.

- Throughout the whole exercise, maintain a back and shoulder position.

- Triceps dips help to build up the triceps muscles at the rear of the upper arms.

Plank

- Begin by doing a push-up with your hands precisely under your shoulders and your toes on the floor.

- Engage your core to maintain a straight line from head to heels.

- Maintaining appropriate form, hold this posture for as long as you can.

- The lower back and abdominal muscles, as well as other core muscles, are the focus of the plank exercise.

Modified Push-Ups

- Start in the push-up posture, but bend your knees to the floor instead of standing on your toes.

- Keep your back straight as you crouch down until your chest is almost touching the ground.

- Regain your original posture by pushing up.

- Modified push-ups assist the upper body while strengthening the chest, shoulders, and triceps.

Step-Ups

- Search for a solid step or platform for step-ups.

- Pushing through the heel, raise the opposite foot after stepping onto the platform with the first.

- Return to the ground with the same foot leading, then repeat with the other foot.

- Step-ups concentrate on the legs' muscles, particularly the quadriceps, hamstrings, and glutes.

A good rule of thumb is to start with resistance or weights suitable for your strength level and then progressively increase the intensity as you advance. Perform each exercise two to three times in sets of ten to fifteen. Allow at least 48 hours between strength-training sessions to ensure muscle recovery.

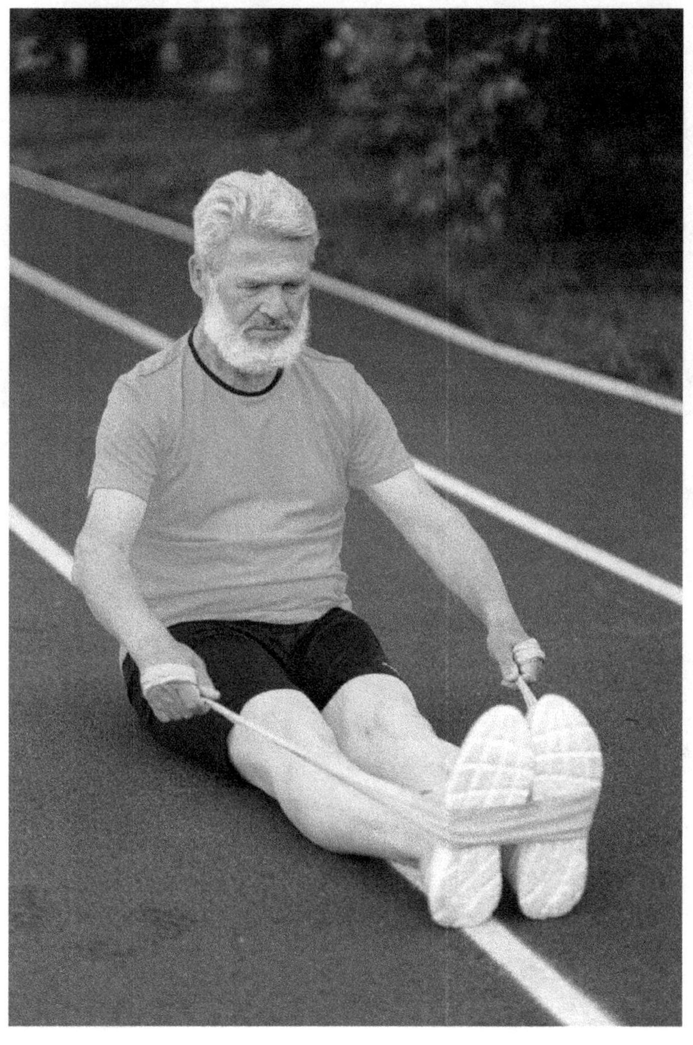

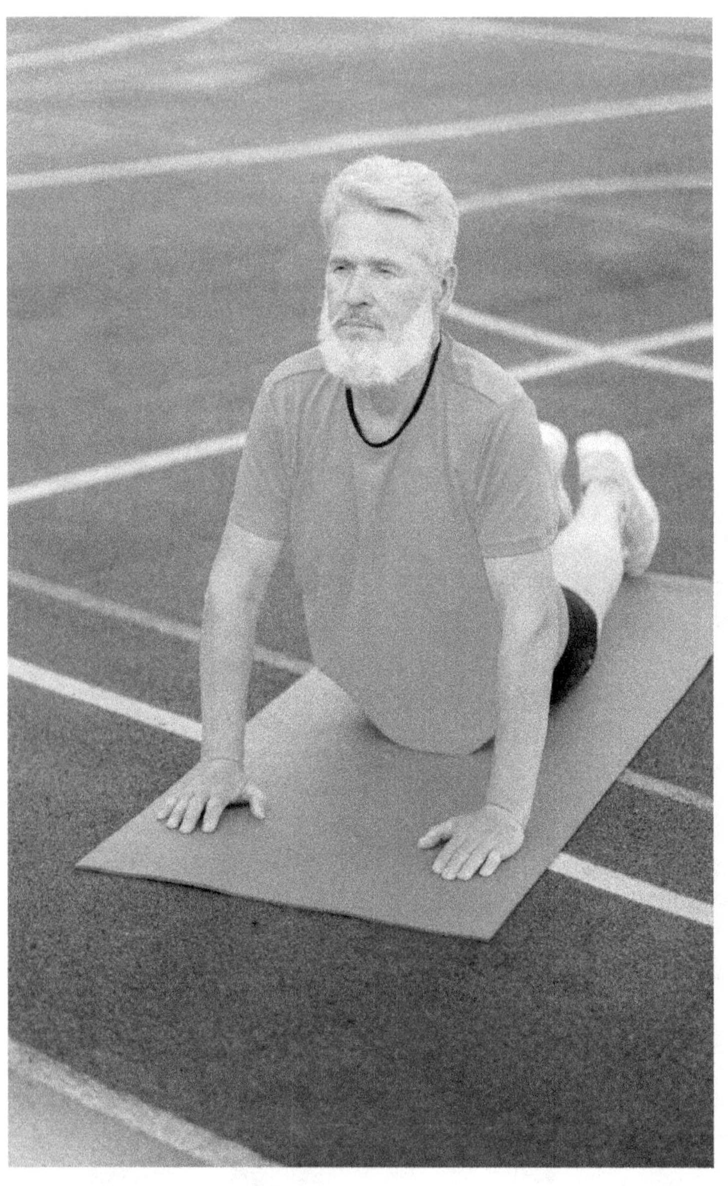

Chapter 8: Cardiovascular Exercise for Seniors

Cardiovascular activity, sometimes called aerobic exercise, is crucial for seniors to keep their hearts healthy, increase their endurance, control their weight, and improve their general well-being. Regular cardiovascular exercise may assist in maintaining a good quality of life and lower the chance of developing chronic conditions. For seniors, the following cardiovascular workouts are suggested:

Walking:

- A low-impact workout that can be performed anytime anyplace is walking.

- Increase the time and intensity gradually, starting at a comfortable speed.

- Try to walk for at least 75 minutes at a robust pace or 150 minutes at a moderate pace per week.

- Cycling is a fantastic, easy-on-the-joint cardiovascular workout.

- If riding outside is not an option, consider utilizing a stationary bike or enrolling in a group cycling class.

- Increase the time and resistance progressively after starting with shorter periods.

- Every muscle in the body is used during swimming, a low-impact activity.

- It may assist in increasing cardiovascular fitness and is accessible to the joints.

- Consider taking water aerobics lessons or learning new swimming techniques to mix up your routine.

Dancing:

- A pleasant and exciting approach to raising your heart rate is through dancing.

- Participate in a dancing class or dance to your favorite music at home.

- It enhances balance, coordination, and cardiovascular stamina.

Tai Chi:

- Deep breathing and soft, flowing movement are combined in the martial art of tai chi.

- Balance, flexibility, and cardiovascular fitness are all enhanced.

- Look for senior-specific Tai Chi sessions or practice online with instructional videos.

Water Aerobics:

- Water aerobics is a low-impact activity done in water to relieve joint tension.

- The resistance of the water provides terrific cardiovascular exercise.

- Join a senior-specific water aerobics class near the pool or community center.

Stationary Exercises:

- Consider utilizing a treadmill, stationary cycle, or elliptical machine if you have restricted mobility or want to work out indoors.

- These devices provide you a cardiovascular exercise while letting you manage the intensity and keep an eye on your heart rate.

- Senior-specific aerobics courses are offered at several fitness facilities and community organizations.

- Such programs as low-impact aerobics, Zumba Gold, or cardio dance courses should be sought out.

- These sessions provide supervised activities that prioritize cardiovascular health while considering the requirements of older citizens.

- Climbing steps is an efficient cardiovascular workout that may be performed at home, in a public space, or on a stair climber machine.

- It gradually increases the time and intensity, starting with a few flights of steps.

Outdoor Activities:

- Take part in outdoor pursuits like gardening, hiking, or sports like tennis or golf.

- These pursuits combine the pleasure of the great outdoors with a cardiovascular workout.

Chapter 9: Balance Exercises for Seniors

Seniors must practice balance exercises to retain independence, increase stability, and avoid falls. Here are some balancing exercises that are suggested for seniors

Single Leg Stands:

- If necessary, use a firm chair or countertop as a support when standing.

- For 30 seconds, lift one leg and maintain balance on the other.

- Repeat while changing legs.

- As you gain experience, try balancing without support or with your eyes closed.

Walk From Heel To Toe:

- Your toes should meet or be just shy of touching when you place the heel of one foot precisely in front of the other.

- Step forward once again with your heel in front of your toes.

- Follow this rhythm of walking for approximately 20 steps.

- If necessary, use a wall or railing to support this exercise.

Leg Raises While Standing:

- Holding onto the chair for support, stand behind it.

- Maintaining a straight knee, extend one leg in front of you.

- Hold the posture for a little while before lowering the leg.

- The other leg, and repeat.

- As you gain experience, attempt completing leg lifts without support.

Yoga Tree Pose

- With your feet together and your arms at your sides, take a tall stance.

- Put all your weight on one foot, then raise the other off the floor.

- Put the elevated foot's sole on the standing leg's inner thigh or calf.

- Bring your hands together in front of your chest after finding your balance.

- For 30 to 60 seconds, maintain this posture.

- On the other side, repeat.

Side leg lifts

- Holding onto the chair for support, stand behind it.

- Keeping the knee straight, extend one leg to the side.

- Hold the posture for a little while before lowering the leg.

- The other leg, and repeat.

- Try executing side leg lifts without holding onto anything as you advance.

Toe Taps

- Holding onto the chair for support, stand behind it.

- While maintaining the leg straight, lift one foot off the ground slightly and tap the toe on the floor sideways.

- Tap the toe forward after bringing the foot back to the center.

- Tap in a forward and side-to-side motion 10 to 15 times on each side.

- Try toe-tapping without hanging onto anything as you advance.

Balancing Wand

- With your arms outstretched in front of you, hold a long wand or stick in each hand.

- Balance on the other leg while raising one leg off the ground.

- Maintain your equilibrium while slowly moving the wand in several directions (up, down, and side to side).

- The other leg, and repeat.

Tai Chi

- Weight-shifting, fluid movements, and regulated breathing are all tai chi exercises that aid balance and coordination.

- Think about enrolling in a Tai Chi class tailored especially for elderly citizens or look for instructional videos online.

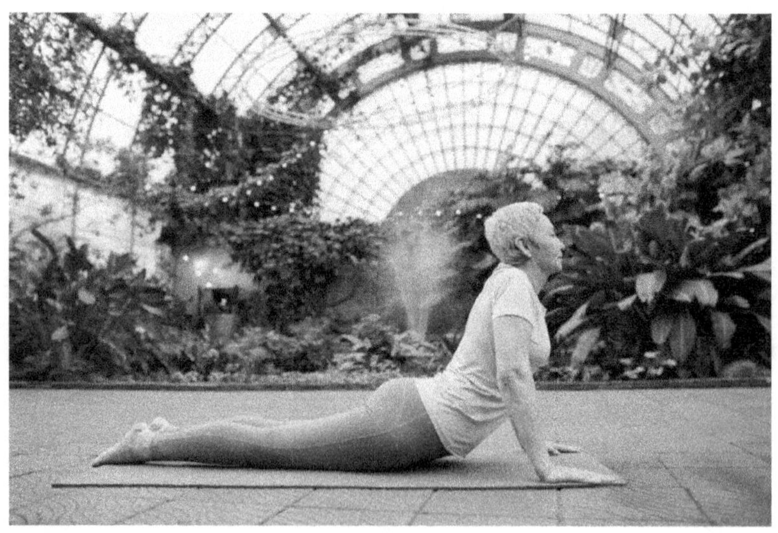

Chapter 10: Improving Flexibility

Increasing flexibility is essential for seniors because it maintains joint mobility, prevents injuries, and improves general physical performance. The following stretching activities are suggested for seniors:

Neck Stretches

- Straighten your spine and shoulders when sitting or standing.

- Gradually lean your head sideways, bringing your ear to your shoulder.

- Follow the stretch for 10 to 15 seconds.

- On the other side, repeat.

- To stretch various neck muscles, make gentle head motions forward and backward.

Shoulders Rolls

- Arms at sides, either standing or sitting.

- Slowly round your shoulders forward.

- Repeat this process 10 to 15 times, then roll them the other way.

- Shoulder rolls aid in releasing tension and enhancing shoulder joint flexibility.

Stretching the arms and chest

- One arm should be extended straight in front of you at shoulder height.

- With your opposite hand, gently bring the outstretched arms fingers back toward your body.

- Follow the stretch for 10 to 15 seconds.

- Continue by using the opposite arm.

- To stretch the chest muscles, stand close to a doorway, press your forearm on the doorframe, and slowly lean forward.

Side bends

- With your feet shoulder-width apart, stand or sit with your arms at your sides.

- Bend sideways and slowly glide one hand down the side of your leg.

- Lean neither forward nor backward while keeping your other arm relaxed.

- Follow the stretch for 10 to 15 seconds.

- On the other side, repeat.

- Side bends increase waist and spine flexibility.

Seated Forward Fold

- Place your feet flat on the ground while perched on the edge of a chair.

- Reach your hands toward the floor or your feet as you slowly bend forward from the hips.

- Keep your shoulders rounded and your back straight.

- Follow the stretch for 10 to 15 seconds.

- The lower back and hamstrings are stretched during the sitting forward fold.

Quadriceps Stretch

- For support, squat close to a chair or wall.

- Bring your foot up toward your glutes while bending one knee.

- Take hold of your ankle or foot with your hand and slowly bring it toward your glutes.

- Hold your knees together while maintaining a straight back.

- Follow the stretch for 10 to 15 seconds.

- The other leg and repeat.

- Stretching the quadriceps may increase the flexibility in the front of the thigh.

Calf Stretches

- Put your hands on the wall in front of you as you stand.

- Step backward with one foot, keeping it straight and the heel firmly planted.

- Feel the rear leg's calf stretch as you gently lean forward.

- Follow the time for 10 to 15 seconds.

- The other leg, and repeat.

- Stretching the calf muscles increase their flexibility.

Ankle circles

- Sit back and firmly place your feet on the ground.

- Lift one foot off the ground, and then gently and circularly rotate the ankle.

- Make 10-15 rounds in one direction before changing to the other.

- Put the other foot down and repeat.

- The ankle joint's flexibility and mobility are enhanced via ankle circles.

Full body stretching

- Put your feet shoulder-width apart and stand tall.

- Spread your arms out before you, fingers entwined with palms facing upward.

- Feel the stretch down the entire side of your body as you lean gently to one side.

- Maintain the stretch.

- Go back to the middle and gently bend forward at the waist, reaching as far as it feels comfortable, preferably near your toes.

- Your lower back and hamstrings should feel stretched.

- Follow the stretch for 10 to 15 seconds.

- Roll up to a standing posture gradually and lower your arms.

Pilates or yoga

- Think about enrolling in a senior-specific yoga or Pilate's class.

- These techniques include a variety of stretches that concentrate on specific muscle groups while also improving general flexibility.

- An experienced coach can help ensure proper form and technique. Before stretching:

- Warm up your muscles by engaging in brief, mild cardiovascular activities like walking or marching in place.

- Avoid jumping or jerking when testing, and focus on moving slowly and softly.

- Never force a stretch or cause discomfort; remember to breathe deeply and relax in each space.

Here are some other pointers to bear in mind while enhancing flexibility:

- To keep your body balanced, evenly stretch both sides.

- Stretching exercises should be a part of your regimen at least 1-2 times a week.

- Be dependable and forgiving. Gains in flexibility require time and consistent practice.

- Observe your body's limitations and pay attention to them. Avoid forcing oneself into positions that are unpleasant or painful.

- Before beginning a new stretching program, speak with your healthcare professional if you have any current medical ailments or concerns.

Increasing your flexibility may significantly improve your range of motion, posture, and general physical well-being as you age. You may maintain or increase your flexibility by including these stretching exercises in your daily routine, enhancing your mobility and quality of life.

Chapter 12: Staying Motivated

It might be challenging to stay motivated to exercise as you age, but with the appropriate techniques and attitude, you can keep your excitement and dedication to your fitness program.

Keep your motivation strong by following these suggestions:

Define Specific, Measurable, Achievable, Relevant, and Time-Bound (SMART) objectives: Next, define realistic and achievable objectives. Specific goals offer you something to work for and keep you motivated and focused. To acknowledge your progress, divide your long-term objectives into more manageable, shorter-term benchmarks.

Choose Exercises and things You Truly like: Find stuff you truly want. You'll likely adhere to your workout schedule if you love the activities you're doing, whether it's yoga, dancing, swimming, or nature walks. Look into many possibilities to see which ones speak to you.

Establish a routine for your workouts and regard them as crucial appointments with yourself: Set out particular hours in your schedule for exercise, and prioritize it. Having a set plan makes it simpler for you to continue with your activities and helps you form a habit.

Change up Your Regimen: Change up your workout regimen to prevent boredom. Include various exercises, try some new ones, or experiment with your workout location. Boredom is avoided by adding diversity and keeping things interesting. Additionally, it puts your body through various difficulties that promote ongoing development.

Find a Workout Partner: Working out with a buddy, or family member, or in a group fitness class may help with accountability and inspiration. When you exercise with others, the activity is more fun, and you are likelier to stick with it. On your fitness adventures, you may support and encourage one another.

Keep a log of your workouts: noting the exercises, length of time, and difficulty level. You can see your accomplishments and how far you've come by keeping track of your progress. It may work as a strong motivator and remind you of the advantages of exercising for your health and well-being.

Milestones should be celebrated: as should your progress. Reward yourself with something significant, such as a little treat or a new fitness-related item, whenever you hit a milestone or accomplish a goal. Honoring your accomplishments strengthens the good emotions connected to exercise and motivates you to keep going.

Keeping a good outlook and focusing on the advantages of regular exercise is essential: Please pay attention to how practice makes you feel, any gains in strength or flexibility you've seen, and how it improves your general health. Be sure to highlight the happiness and achievement the exercise gives.

Be Flexible and Adaptive: There may be days when maintaining your usual schedule is difficult due to unanticipated events or private obligations.

Be adaptive and flexible. Find other methods to remain active, even if it's for a shorter period if you can't stick to your regular exercise schedule. Always keep in mind that something is always preferable to nothing.

Seek Support and Stay Informed: Surround yourself with a network of friends, family, or fitness experts who can support you and inspire you. Keep up with the most recent fitness fads, health advice, and senior-specific fitness regimens. Knowing your alternatives might help you stay interested and motivated.

Keep in mind that it's common for motivation to change over time. When you lack motivation, remind yourself of your objectives, consider the advantages of exercise, and start small. Celebrate your accomplishments, maintain your commitment, and take pleasure in the road to a healthier and more active way of life.

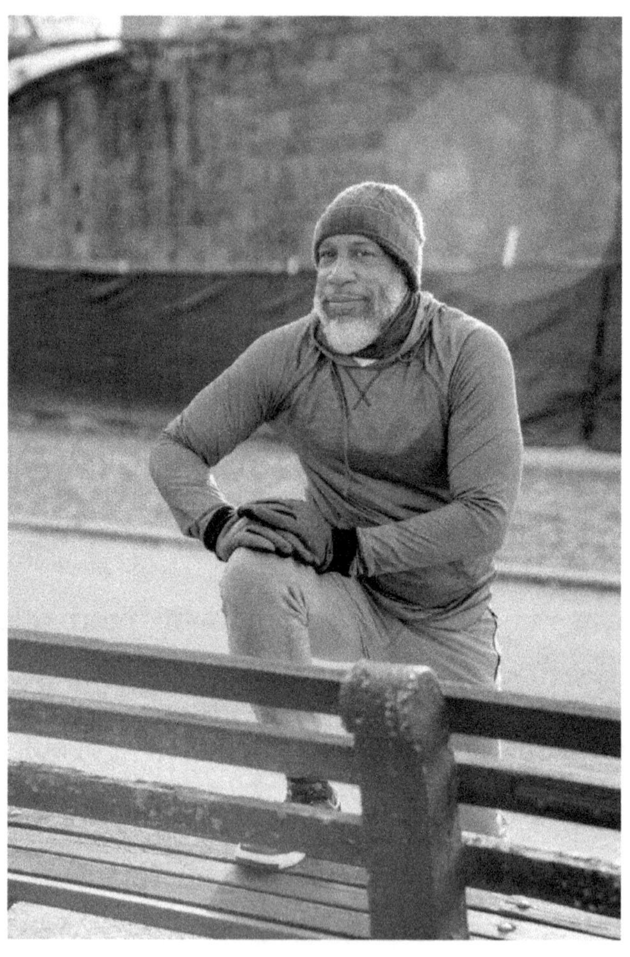

Conclusion

Seniors benefit greatly from exercise, which has several physical, psychological, and emotional advantages. It is always possible to start an exercise program, and seniors may enhance their mobility, general health, and quality of life with the appropriate direction and attitude.

Seniors may focus on various fitness goals by including multiple activities in their program. Stretching exercises keep muscles loose and avoid muscular tightness. At the same time, cardiovascular workouts improve heart health and endurance, strength training increases and maintains muscle mass, flexibility exercises promote joint mobility, and balancing exercises lower the chance of falling.

Individual fitness levels must be considered when creating an exercise program, as well as realistic objectives and fun, long-lasting exercises. To avoid injuries and encourage long-term commitment, it's essential to advance gradually, use appropriate techniques, and pay attention to your body.

Seniors may overcome obstacles and remain devoted to their fitness regimen by establishing objectives, choosing pleasant activities, developing a timetable, monitoring their progress, getting assistance, and having a good attitude.

Seniors who exercise regularly may age gracefully, remain independent, and have busy, satisfying lives. Accepting the advantages of exercise and prioritizing it can improve physical health, confidence, mood, and general well-being.

Remember that prioritizing your health is always early enough. Start working out right now and allow the transformational power of exercise to lead you to a senior life that is healthier, happier, and more active.

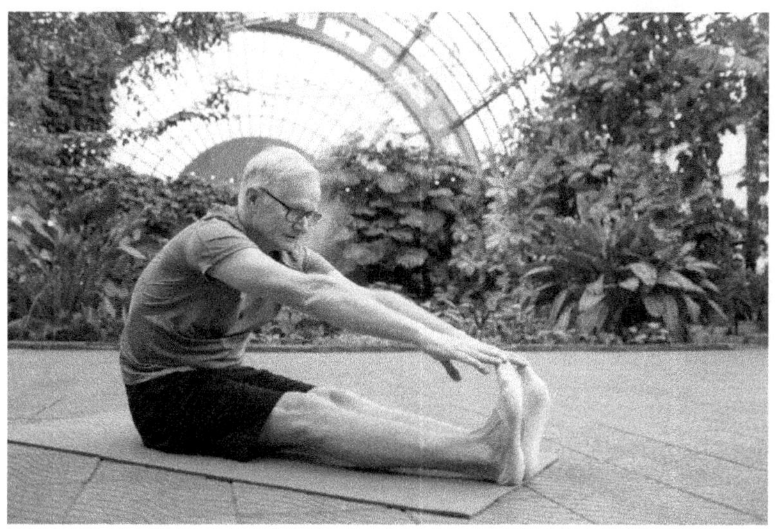